Pebble Theatre
for the young performer

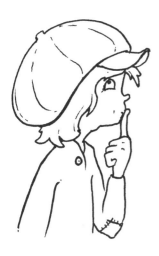
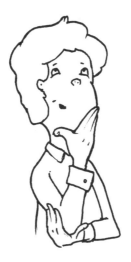
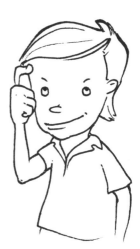

A book for intrepid, interesting, and imaginative children to connect with other talented and creative young people through the art of performing.

In today's world of overwhelming uses of technology with heavily scheduled days, we sometimes lack the face to face conversations, and we miss the value in the sharing of laughter. We all need to take time to imagine, daydream and reflect. And, it is imperative, that we appreciate the value of the arts in the lives of all of our children!

This book is dedicated to all the delightful children, supportive parents, and talented adult volunteers who shared their music, art, and theatre knowledge, throughout the many years to make the experiences of the Ellensburg Children's Musical Theatre possible.

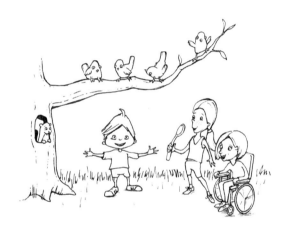

Published in the United States by Bill Sweeney Design
http://www.billsweeneydesign.com

First American Edition
ISBN: 978-0-692-32590-2

http://www.pebbletheatre.org

Table of Contents:

A note from Donna Nylander 5

Contributors 6

Are you ready? 7

    Pretend and Dramatize 8

    Who? Where? What? 14

    What in the world can we do? Types of theatrical fun 16

Where Can I Look for Ideas? See You at the Library! 39

Backyard Theatre 45

Costumes and Props 51

    A Costume Exercise Just for Fun 53

Stage Directions 55

Moving Beyond the Basics 57

Ice Breakers - Get Things Going 59

Creating Improvisation 63

    Creating Mystery Theatre 76

Final Thoughts - Thank you! 83

Biographies for the Contributors 85

Certificate 90

A Pebble Tossed into the Water

A note from Donna Nylander
Playwright and Director of Ellensburg Children's Musical Theatre

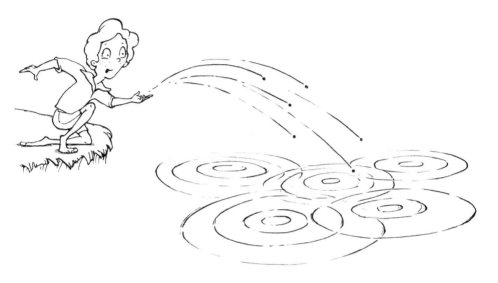

In the summer of 1976, I met with David Blodgett who had just been hired as the first Director of the newly formed Ellensburg Community Schools Program. I shared a script I had written for a children's play, called The Wis Wis Forest. He encouraged me to produce it under the new Community Schools Program. Dr. Russell Ross, a professor at Central Washington University, agreed to compose all the music. Local artists, musicians, teachers, carpenters, actors, moms and dads volunteered to help. The turnout was amazing. We performed an additional weekend because so many people were turned away the first weekend. Thus was the beginning of The Ellensburg Children's Musical Theatre.

I enjoy writing plays that are fun for children, as well as educational and meaningful for the whole audience. For instance, The Light Within, our 2013 production, encouraged children to find the "light" that is his or hers and then share it with others.

A summer program called Pebble Theatre, was established many years ago to encourage children to create their own plays with their siblings and friends. During the week, children learned basics about acting, costumes, plot development, and sharing the stage. In small groups, a plot was developed, roles were decided, and later they performed for participants and their parents. A pebble tossed into the water will create a circle. A handful of pebbles will create many circles that intersect and connect. Thus developed the philosophy for Pebble Theatre, for when children connect with other children they make a much bigger splash.

I asked a few Ellensburg Children's Musical Theatre members to help write a book so you can enjoy your own dramatic fun. We hope that together we can inspire talented young people to share their light through creating their own Pebble Theatre.

Who contributed to it?

Donna Nylander, Josephine Yaba Camarillo, Olivia Sweeney, Marian Gerrits, Evan Powell, Kendra Munroe, Justin Gibbens, Debbie Vosburgh, Nomi Pearce, and Bill Sweeney

Are you ready?

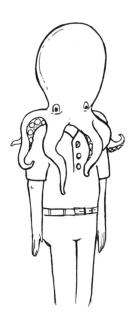

Do you enjoy performing? Well, don't wait until another performance "happens." YOU can create your own event! This book is our invitation to you to create your own Pebble Theatre and we hope it will inspire you. We will ask you questions to get you thinking about who you want to include, offer ideas on where you can make something happen, and give you suggestions for possible types of dramatic fun you can choose. We offer a list of books that can give you ideas for poems or stories to act out. Check out the list of household items that you can use to make costumes and props. We even offer an original script based on silly nursery rhymes for a Reader's Theatre event. For those looking for backyard fun there is a chapter on how to get started. For advanced fun we have included a section on ice breakers, improvisation techniques and games, and writing your own mystery theatre.

Pretend and Dramatize

Deciding when, where, what and why to perform is a fun process. Using one's body and voice to create the audience's belief in the character is the most fun of all! A character is who you become on stage. An actor is the person who plays that character. If you want to be an actor then you need to practice some ways to convince others of your character and story.

First, look around

Good actors are good observers. Wherever or whenever you have the opportunity to watch anyone, of any age or background, watch the face to see how the face gives you information. Do the eyes look happy, sad, angry, interested, or scared. What clues do you get from the person's body? Is the head down? Or held high? Are the shoulders down? Or held back? What position are the arms in? Are they folded across the chest? Are the hands together? Are the hands behind the back? Is one hand resting on the chin? What about the legs or feet? Are the legs together with the feet flat on the floor? Are the feet crossed at the ankles? Are the legs spread apart? Is one foot on the floor and the other in a different position?

What you are observing is called body language. **Body language** includes facial expression, gestures, posture and movement. A good actor uses the face and body to help tell the story with the use of body language.

Find a mirror. Watch yourself in the mirror as you change the position of your body and facial expressions such as the eyes and mouth for different kinds of feelings. How does your face look when you are happy? Surprised? Confused? Sleepy? How do you show your body posture to match your face? You may have friends join you so you can take turns interpreting each other's feelings.

You can tell a story without a voice, just by pretending. Pretending is when you act or speak to make something seem like it is happening, but it is not. Have you ever pretended that you were sleeping when you weren't? If so, you already know how to pretend!

Pretend you are in a house.
How does an audience know you are in a house? You could pretend to read a book. You could pretend to watch television. You could pretend to eat something. How would the audience know what you are doing?

Pretend you are going outside.
How does an audience know you are going outside? You could pretend to put on a hat and coat and mittens. That would show it is winter and cold. You could you put on sun screen and sunglasses. That would show it is summer and sunny.

Pretend you are walking through a door.
Is it a regular kind of door? Or is it a sliding door? How do you show the difference? What do you do when you get outside?

Do you make a snowball? Snowman? Slide? Skate? Experience cold? How do you show what is happening? Is it warm? Do you find shade? Do you go for a walk? A bike ride? Swim? Sun bathe?

So you see how your actions alone can tell your story. You are using only your body language to tell or actually show your story. If you are with friends have them create simple actions and facial expression that will tell their story.

Here are a few pretend stories to practice. Do not use voices. Tell your story with your face and body and action.

You are home alone.
What are you doing? Reading? Watching TV? Talking on the phone? Checking your email?

The door bell rings.
Who is at the door? A pizza delivery? Do you have money to pay? Is it a friend and now the two of you will have pizza? Use your actions to show us the entire story.

What other possibilities could there be? Perhaps a mailman? Why does the mailman ring your door bell? Could UPS have a package? If so, how do you let us know what is in the package? Maybe the person at the door just found your dog. Was your dog lost? Was your dog hurt?

You are in a dark woods.
Are you alone or is someone with you? If so, who?

Now what happens? Thunder? Lightening? A strange animal? A lost child?

What do you do? What is the result of what you do? Remember no voices.

Your actions and body language tells the story.

You find a box.

Where are you when you discover the box? How big or little, heavy or light is the box? What is its shape? Does it have a smell? Are there any sounds coming from the box? What do you discover about the box? How do you discover what is in the box, and how does your body language let the audience learn what is in the box? Do you need anyone or any tool to help with telling the story of the box?

You and your friends may want to create other scenes (or scenarios) for each other to act out. You and your friends can write the ideas for the scenarios down on small pieces of paper. Then place the papers in a hat or basket. Ask each of your friends to close their eyes and reach in and pick one piece of paper. We call that **drawing a paper**. The idea written on the piece of paper that each one draws becomes the idea that person will dramatize. Only the basic idea has been written down. The actor fully develops the idea and acts it out in body language with acting only.

So for example: "You go to get your bicycle and something is wrong."

Now the actor must turn that idea into the story, demonstrated with body language actions. The actor must create the story with body language in order to tell: Where is the bike located? At home? At school? In front of store? What is wrong with the bicycle? What does the person need to do to solve the problem? How does the actor show us how the problem was or wasn't solved.

Adding emotion, a little chuckle and a tear

Pretend something funny just happened. Start smiling, then make a little laugh, then a bigger laugh, then start laughing really hard! Then laugh so hard you are rolling on the floor with laughter!!!

Next, pretend that something sad just happened. Look sad, then wipe pretend tears away, add a little cry, then cry harder, then sink to the floor crying really, really hard. Now reverse the crying, until you are barely whimpering, Next wipe your pretend tears away and slowly begin to smile until you have a broad smile.

Time to speak up

Now let's see how your voice can add to help a character become larger, and more significant. The same words can be said in many different ways.

1) Pretend you have a friend walking to school, but he or she is far ahead of you.

   Shout these words: "Hey, Joe, (or Josephine), I have something really important to tell you!"

2) Pretend you are in a dark and scary room, and whisper to your friend: "Hey, Joe, (or Josephine), I have something really important to tell you!"

3) Pretend, that for some reason, you are very angry with your

friend: "Hey, Joe (or Josephine) I have something really important to tell you!"

4) Finally, pretend that what you want to share is really funny. So start laughing or giggling and try to get the words out: "Hey, Joe, (or Josephine) I have something really important to tell you!"

When you were doing these little pretend scenes, did you remember to match, your face and body language to your words? If you did, then you are on your way to becoming a great actor!

A note to all those who are watching: Please applaud!

Peripheral Vision

The ability to see things to the side without looking directly at them is called **peripheral vision**. Lift your arms out from your sides. Look straight ahead of you. Wiggle your fingers as you bring your hands closer together. Now move them back to your sides until you don't see them anymore. Notice how you can see your fingers wiggle and then as they move farther back - then they are gone! You use peripheral vision at school, in gym class, when you play football, when you ride a bike, when you dance, or on the stage!

Pretend you are on the stage. Look straight ahead at the person speaking. Without moving your eyes what do you see on each side of your body? Can you see furniture, other people, actions to either side of you?

Now pretend something is going to happen on another part

of the stage. You are supposed to be surprised, but in order to react you need to know when that "something" happens. So you must use your peripheral vision.

Who do want to ask to join you?

- sister or brother
- cousins
- aunts or uncles
- grandparent
- parent or step-parent
- best friends
- someone you want to know better
- neighborhood kids
- friend from school
- with club group (scouts, youth group, 4H)
- babysitter
- classroom
- who else do you know?

Where could your Pebble Theater happen?

- in your living room
- in your family room
- in your carport
- in your garage
- in your driveway
- on a patio
- on a porch
- in a backyard

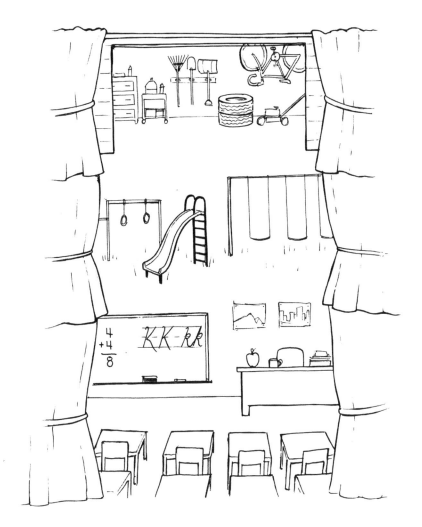

- among some trees
- near playground equipment
- in a park
- in your playhouse
- in a tree house
- at a day care center
- in your school or classroom

- at a retirement home or skilled nursing facility
- at your place of worship
- at a community center
- in the windows of a store, downtown or in a mall

What in the World Can We Do? Types Theatrical Fun

- Create a talent show.
- Create a backyard drama camp.
- Create a mystery theatre for a birthday party.
- Create fun and crazy improvisations.
- Read and dramatize poetry.
- Dramatize a historical moment in history.
- Dramatize a story or fable from another country.
- Dramatize a Native American legend.
- Dramatize a fairy tale (you could invent a new ending).
- Dramatize a story from your religion.
- Dramatize classical music or words to a contemporary song.
- Dramatize an original story.

Which of these have you done before? Which of these do want you want to try?

Want a little more information on each type of performance? Here you go!

Talent Show

A fun program could be a talent show. This program can be easily put together with siblings, relatives, neighbors, school buddies, or church friends. You can put the program together

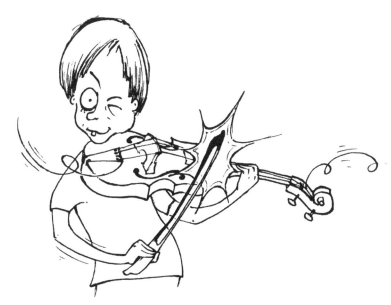

for a family gathering, holiday gathering, your classroom, a school program, a summer fun day, or special program for a retirement home or nursing facility.

Make a list of children you know who have talent. The talent may be in music, reciting poetry, or telling a joke, or any of the many things listed in other parts of this book.

When you become aware of a talented person, save the correct spelling of the person's the name, a phone number, and an email address. Keep the information in a special notebook or in your phone. If a piano is needed but not available you may want to borrow a keyboard. If you use a keyboard, you will need to check for available electricity.

When you have chosen all of your participants, you may wish to have a meeting and choose a date, time, and place to perform. If you choose a nursing home or nursing facility you

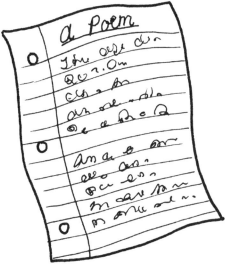

will need to contact them to ask for an appointment to tell them of your idea. Ask to see the room where you would be performing.

Reading poetry and dramatization

There are many fun and funny contemporary poets. Some poets give insight into things in our lives. Other well known poets of other centuries are revered and studied in classes today. Who is your audience going to be? Younger or older? Will your audience be folks you know, an audience of all ages or backgrounds? Knowing who your audience is will help to determine whom you may choose for your poet/poets. Page 40 has suggested poets.

To dramatize means to act something out in a way that tells a story. When you are on stage you need to tell the story with your voice and body.

You may choose to have one or several good voices read the poetry with others performing the poem. Some readers may want to perform as they recite. It is best to encourage your readers/speakers to have the poetry memorized. The audience will enjoy the program more if there is eye contact with them. Eye contact is when you can look into the eyes of the audience. It can be short, but it let's them know you see them!

Dramatize an historical moment in history

You could honor a person and highlight that person's contribution to others, such as the genius of Alexander Graham Bell, the intrepid Helen Keller and imaginative Annie Sullivan. Do you want to inform your audience about a specific event in history? It may be the anniversary of the trip to the   moon, or the creation of laws to protect the rights of children. You may wish to highlight the Lewis and Clark expedition. You may wish to make a difference in social behavior by creating a story about bullying or developing a new friendship. The accidental creation of the beloved Teddy Bear, the invention of the simple wooden pencil, or our useful crayons are all interesting stories for children. There are many possibilities.

Dramatize a Native American legend

The Native American stories are rich in drama and imaginative in content. The stories were told to help the children to learn the history of their people, and to explain the world around them. Stories can explain the relationship between people and animals, seasons of the year, the importance of water, or the rotation of the earth and its relationship to the moon. When dramatizing a Native American legend, one does not want to change or embellish the story out of respect for the traditional legend. To enhance the performance one may wish to use a drum or wooden flute, or other sound effects for animals, birds, rain, or thunder.

Dramatize a fairy tale

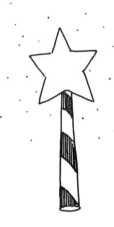

Many fairy tales are well known. Dramatizations are a fun way to revisit those stories, but there are many fairy tales that are less well known that are delightful and can be enjoyed by any audience. What would happen if The Three Little Pigs were in opera style? Do you have books on the shelf that are favorites? Go to your library and look for a great fairy tale, or a book of fables (such as Aesop's Fables) and start reading.

Dramatize a story from your religion

Are there stories well known or lesser known that give meaningful information or lessons of life to children? Stories of your religious heritage can lend themselves to dramatization. Ask your religious leader for suggestions to help get you started. This project could enhance a special day and also give significant memories to all the participants.

Dramatize a script already written

Check your library for books with scripts. Also check a second-hand store, such as Goodwill or St. Vincent's. Sometimes children's magazines have scripts in them, and very old school books also have scripts in the text books.

Dramatize music

Music lends itself to creating stories. What do you listen to? Classical, country, pop, or patriotic. Take time to sit with your eyes closed and listen to the music. What is your vision as you listen to the music? Can you create a story for the music with actions? Sometimes songs tell a story with the lyrics or words. Can you dramatize the words? You may do it seriously or do it with humor.

Dramatize an original story

Do you have a story that you have created or written that you would like to have become a play? Is it possible to give it life by dramatizing the story? Does it have a beginning, middle, and end that state the problem, then tells how the problem gets worked out, and then tells of the result of solving the problem?

Dramatize a family story or a fable from another country

All of our ethnic and heritage backgrounds contain rich stories that are informative and dramatic. Are there stories in your own family history that you wish to share? See page 43 for additional story ideas.

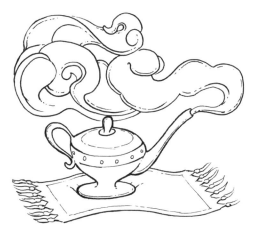

Dramatize Using Shadow Puppets (finger/hand)

Do you know a child confined to a bed or wheelchair, temporarily or for an extended period of time? Here is an idea for you.

Set up a lamp or flashlight in a darkened room. Begin with some very simple movements of hand/finger puppets between the source of light and a flat surface such as a wall or door. Move your hand and fingers around to explore the shape you want. Two hands can make a butterfly, one hand with two fingers up can make a bunny. Now give your puppet a character and voice - is it a young creature with a squeaky voice? Is it an old wise creature with a deep, slow voice?

If you have never been introduced to shadow (fingers/hands) puppets check out a book from the library. Another resource could be an older person, such as a grandparent, neighbor, or older friend. At one time children had few toys with which to play. They often entertained themselves with finger/hand shadow puppets.

After you have introduced and demonstrated your shadow puppets using your fingers and hands, work together to create several shadow puppets. Be creative. Be bold!

When you have created four or five shadow puppet characters create an imaginative story that will include the characters you have both created. Together, as you tell the story, you both will have your shadow puppets perform. If a classmate is confined to a bed, ask the teacher if your class can create some shadow puppets and a story to present to the child who is confined. Perhaps two or three children can ask if they can visit the child with the "surprise."

Some folks may wish to create one-dimensional, flat, cardboard, paper, or stick puppets to use for the shadow puppets. This can be fun too. However, the finger/hand shadow puppet possibilities are more simple and more easily created by a bored or confined young person.

Dramatize a Window Pantomime

In large cities, major department stores often spend thousands of dollars creating magical moving window displays during the Christmas holidays. For small towns there are stores that would enjoy having magical window entertainment. Make a plan for a window pantomime, then approach store owners with your idea. Furniture stores and mattress stores with large windows are frequently and easily accessible, but toy stores and children's clothing stores are also good selections. Sometimes you can find an empty building with great windows. A building owner is usually pleased to draw interest to his/her store. These dramatizations using interpretive music offer possibilities. There are no words used and no "mouthing or lip moving" of words. Faces, body language, and emotions tell the story.

Find classical music that can be interpreted by telling a story through drama. If you do not have knowledge of classical music, talk to your school music teacher or band or orchestra teacher, or a piano teacher for suggestions. Libraries often have a good selection of music you can check out with no charge. Listen to the music and imagine a story that can be told with the music, drama, and costumes.

Here are some ideas that have worked and can inspire you:
- Elves at work in Santa's workshop. Santa falls asleep. What happens?

- A birthday or holiday party for a small group of children. They bring presents. One present is totally inappropriate or wrong. What is the present? What is wrong with it? Is it a funny inappropriate gift? Had they drawn names?

- A large family gathering. What is the composition of the family? Parents, grandparents, aunts, uncles, siblings, babies, a blind family member, a person in a wheelchair, an unexpected guest (if so, who?), an unusual gift (if so, what?). Are there any pets involved? What is the best Christmas present? A parent in uniform shows up unexpectedly. A mom with a tiny baby appears? Santa Claus shows up?

After you get your music story ready, practice several times so you know how it works. Find a store that will be enthusiastic to have you perform.

Each pantomime can last five to ten minutes. The audience is standing outside the window, watching. The music is outside the windows, but the actors are well rehearsed and can hear the music well enough to perform in sync with the music. Some stores can play the music inside and outside the store at the same time.

Have the performers enter the window display area and take positions and freeze. Music begins and performers begin to tell the story. When the story is finished the actors freeze; then, on cue they all stand, take a bow, and exit. One child should remain behind with a large sign that says, "Next performance in 30 minutes" or whatever works for you. (This allows the children to go to the bathroom, get a drink, and think about how to improve his/her performance.)

On any one day you may plan to do two, at most three, performances. The information regarding performances must have signs in the window for at least a week in advance, telling of the plan, with the date and time highlighted.

If free newspaper coverage is possible take advantage of that. Have your family and friends share on social media. Encourage family and friends to come too!

Reader's Theatre

This is a fun example of how you can do simple programs with your friends. Choose some of your friends to either memorize or read the following nursery rhymes. Use voices, body language, and facial expressions to emphasize the lines. Everyone may sit on stools. A variety of heights or styles can be more interesting for the audience. On some lines the actor may stand, or may jump up suddenly. Some actors may want to move about to emphasize words, shake a fist, point a finger, smile, scowl, or giggle with the lines. You can interpret the lines or words with your voice to give your audience more enjoyment. The more energy you invest in the presentation the more fun your audience will have. You may add to the presentation by taking a large brown grocery bag, cut up one middle side, cut out holes for your arms, turn inside out, and each one has a vest. Use crayons or felt-tip markers for design. You could also use large white plastic garbage bags to make vests.

The Nursery Rhyme Spoof by Donna Nylander

Write the name of who's speaking on the line.

_____ Baa, baa, black sheep have you any wool?
Yes, sir, yes, sir, three bags full!
One for my master and one for my dame,
But none for the little boy who cries down the lane!
Is that okay?

_____ Well, what was the reason, I mean why, was the little
boy crying down the lane?

_____ We don't know, do we?

_____ The black sheep decided not to give the little boy
any wool. I mean, the statement was, "And none for
the little boy that cries down the lane."
That isn't okay.

_____ Just because he was crying is not a good enough
reason for not giving him any wool. The black
sheep needs to go down the lane and find out why
the little boy was crying.

_____ Right!

___All___ Not okay!

_____ Tom, Tom, the piper's son
Stole a pig and away he run.
The pig was eat and Tom was beat and
Tom went crying down the street!

_____ No, that is not okay.

_____ Tom should not have stolen the pig.

_____ And he should not have run.

_____ But then it says, "The pig was eat. " Who did that?

_____ That was wrong.

_____ And Tom was beat.

_____ Definitely wrong!

_____ And Tom went crying down the street.

_____ NO WONDER!

___All___ It's not okay.

_____ Jack be nimble, Jack be quick.
Jack jumped over the candlestick.
Is that okay?

_____ Well, we don't know if the candle was lit when he
jumped over the candlestick.

_____ If the candle was lit, then no matter how nimble
Jack was, he should not have jumped over the
candlestick.

___All___ It's not okay.

_____ Simple Simon met a pie man going to the fair.
Said Simple Simon to the pie man, let me taste your
ware.
Said the pie man to Simple Simon, show me first

your penny.
Said Simple Simon to the pie man,
Indeed, I have not any.
Is that okay?

_____ Is that okay? Well, the pie man was cautious. I
mean, he wasn't going to give Simple Simon pie
without first seeing the penny. But, on the other
hand, what we don't know is, had Simple Simon
had anything to eat that day? Maybe he was really
hungry. In that case…

_____ (interrupting) You are right. The pie man should
have given at least a piece of the pie to Simple
Simon.

_____ I would have.

_____ Got to look at the profits, though. Got to look at the
bottom line.

_____ The bottom line is, Simple Simon may have been
very, very hungry.

___All___ It's not okay.

_____ Sing a song of sixpence, a pocket full of rye.
Four and twenty blackbirds baked in a pie.
When the pie was opened the birds began to sing.
Wasn't that a dainty dish to set before the king?
The king was in the counting house counting out
his money.
The queen was in the parlor eating bread and honey.

The maid is in the garden hanging out the clothes
And along came a blackbird and snipped off her nose!

_____ Is that okay?

_____ No, that is not okay. Even if the birds were going to
sing, that certainly is not a dainty dish to set before
anyone, even a king. And the queen eating bread
and honey, okay, but did she know what happened
to the maid? They snipped off her nose?

___All___ That is not okay.

_____ London Bridge is falling down, falling down, falling
down.
London Bridge is falling down, my fair lady!
Take the keys and lock her up, lock her up, lock her up!

_____ Take the keys and lock her up, my fair lady!
Is that okay?

_____ Wait a minute! Because London Bridge is falling
down, then we have to lock up my fair lady?

_____ No way! Just because the bridge is falling down is
not a reason for locking up my fair lady.

_____ Unless of course she was the engineer who
designed the bridge.

_____ And we have no evidence of that!

___All___ Not okay!

_____ Mary had a little lamb, its fleece was white as snow,
And everywhere that Mary went the lamb was sure to go.
It followed her to school one day, which was against the rules,
And made the children laugh and play to see a lamb at school!
Is that okay?

_____ Really, it probably was okay that the lamb followed her to school one day. Cats and dogs do it all the time.

_____ But here is the problem. When the children laughed and played, you know, they played that they were little lambs and followed Mary around going baaaa baaaa, and it, well, it made her feel embarrassed and she cried. The children should not have teased her!

___All___ That is not okay!

_____ Old Mother Hubbard went to her cupboard
To get her poor dog a bone.
And when she got there, the cupboard was bare
And so the poor dog had none.
Is that okay?

___All___ That is not okay.

_____ Jack and Jill went up the hill to fetch a pail of water.

Jack fell down and broke his crown and Jill came tumbling after.
Is that okay?

_____ Well, no. Jack and Jill went up the hill to fetch a pail of water. Okay. It sounds okay. But then, when Jack fell down and broke his crown, and Jill came tumbling after, there was no adult to check over Jack's crown or to see if Jill was really okay. Adults were neglectful.

___All___ That's not okay.

_____ Little Miss Muffet sat on a tuffet eating her curds and whey.
Along came a spider and sat down beside her and frightened Miss Muffet away.
Is that okay?
Let's see now, did I get this right?

_____ Little Miss Muffet is sitting on a tuffet, right?

_____ Yes.

_____ And along came a spider and sat down beside her. On the tuffet?

_____ Well, I guess so.

_____ Did he declare his intentions? Did he just want to sit beside her, or did he want her curds and whey?

_____ With the information that has been given to us, we don't really know, do we?

_____ If the spider had wanted my curds and whey I would have said, "Have at them. " I hate curds and whey, and my mother knows that, too!

_____ There was an old woman who lived in a shoe.
She had so many children she did not know what to do.
So she gave them some broth without any bread And whipped them all soundly and sent them to bed.
Is that okay?

_____ She gave them some broth without any bread.
That's okay. Because with so many children, maybe that's all she had. But to whip them all soundly and send them to bed?

___All___ (emphatically) That is not okay!

_____ Peter, Peter, pumpkin eater had a wife and couldn't keep her.
He put her in a pumpkin shell…

___All___ (interrupting) That's not okay! (shouting) No further discussion needed.

_____ Diddle, diddle, dumpling, my son John Went to bed with one shoe on.

_____ Is that okay?

_____ He went to bed with one shoe on?

_____ That's okay.

_____ He probably was very sleepy.

_____ And if he doesn't do it every night, no big deal!

___All___ It's okay!

_____ Rock a bye baby in the tree top.
When the wind blows the cradle will rock.
When the bough breaks the cradle will fall
And down will come baby, cradle and all!
Is that okay?

_____ Definitely not! First of all, who put the cradle in the
tree top and how high was that tree?

_____ And when the wind began to blow, no one
checked on the cradle? It must have been a big
wind to break the bough and, with the cradle falling
and all, where were the adults?

___All___ Definitely NOT okay!!

_____ Hey, diddle diddle, the cat and the fiddle.
The cow jumped over the moon.
The little dog laughed to see such a sight
And the dish ran away with the spoon.
Is that okay?

_____ Well, let's see now. The dish ran away with the
spoon. Is that okay? And the little dog laughed

to see such a sight. Is that okay? But then did he notify anyone? How about the fork and the knife? Did he tell them?

_____ And the cow jumping over the moon? Did that curdle the milk?

_____ Whose cow was she anyway? Could she do that again? (enthusiastically)

_____ I wonder.

_____ Sorry, we don't have enough information.

_____ Hickory, dickory, dock, the mouse ran up the clock.
The clock struck one; the mouse ran down.
Hickory, dickory, dock.
Is that okay?

_____ Now just a minute. When that clock struck one, and the mouse ran down, no one ever tells where the mouse ran to.

_____ Without knowing where the mouse ran after it ran down…

_____ We need more information about where the mouse ran to.

_____ So it's not okay?

___All___ It is not okay.

_____ Three little kittens lost their mittens and they began

to cry.
Oh, Mommy dear, we greatly fear our mittens we
have lost.
What, lost your mittens? You naughty kittens!
Then you shall have no pie!
Is that okay?

_____ Really, you can't blame the mother cat, "Mommy
Dear," for being so upset with the three little kittens
losing their mittens! Not just one mitten, not just
one kitten. Three kittens lost both mittens. I think it
was okay to tell them that they shall have no pie.

_____ They could go look for the mouse that ran down
from the clock!

_____ Humpty Dumpty sat on a wall.
Humpty Dumpty had a great fall.
All the king's horses and all the king's men
Couldn't put Humpty Dumpty together again.
Is that okay?

_____ It is pretty pathetic that all the king's horses and
all the king's men couldn't put Humpty Dumpty
together again!

_____ Not really okay.

_____ They could have tried a glue gun!

_____ Georgie porgie, pudding and pie
Kissed the girls and made them cry.

_____All_____ It's not okay…not anymore! (loud cheers)

_____ The queen of hearts she made some tarts
All on a summer's day.
The knave of hearts he stole the tarts
And took them clean away.

_____ The queen had worked very hard making the tarts.

_____ The knave should not have stolen the tarts!

_____All_____ It is not okay!

_____ Old King Cole was a merry old soul
And a merry old soul was he!
He called for his pipe and he called for his bowl
And he called for his fiddlers three.
Every fine fiddler had a fine fiddle and a very nice
fiddle had he.
Tweedle dum tweedle dee went the fiddlers three.
Tweedle dum tweedle dee dee deedle dee.
Is that okay?

_____ Well, sure it is okay. If he likes that kind of music. It
isn't exactly the kind of music I like to listen to. I
mean tweedle dumdedumdeedeedle dee. Not my
kind of music. However, different kinds of music
make our lives more interesting.
I guess…

_____ Star light, star bright; first star I see tonight.

I wish I may, I wish I might have the wish I wish tonight.
I wish all children big and small
Not know hunger and not know fear.
But a caring adult is always near!
I wish all children big and small
Feel loved and valued most of all.

(Sometimes we do things or say things that are really hurtful. With the nursery rhymes, the speakers were telling us that some things are just not okay!)

Notes:

Where can you look for ideas? See you at the Library!

by Josephine Yaba Camarillo

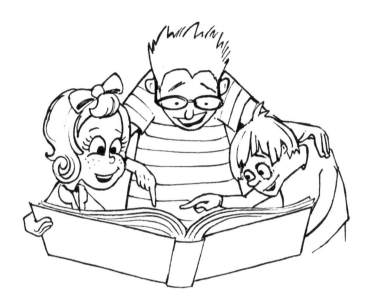

Children's Poets that Work for Performance

The works of the following poets are great examples that can easily turn into a fun performance piece. With the use of props, tone of voice, exaggerated actions and music, any poem can take on a new life. Be creative! Think about what the poem is saying, what is happening, and how you can show the audience with your voice, words, and actions. Don't be shy to overreact or under react, depending on the poem. This point is to REACT! Use body language and voice inflection.

Shel Silverstein

- Everything on it: poems and drawings (2011)
- Runny Babbit: a billy sook (2005)
- Where the sidewalk ends (1974)

Jack Prelutsky

- Be glad your nose is on your face and other poems: some of the best of Jack Prelutsky (2008)
- A pizza the size of the sun: poems (1996)
- The new kid on the block: poems (1984)

Calef Brown

- Soup for Breakfast: poems and pictures (2008)
- Flamingos on the roof (2006)
- We Go Together (2013)

Karen Jo Shapiro

- I must go down to the beach again and other poems (2007)
- Because I could not stop my bike: and other poems (2003)

Jeff Moss

- The other side of the door: poems (1991)
- The butterfly jar (1989)

Kenn Nesbitt

- The tighty whitey spider: and more wacky animal poems I totally made up (2010)
- My hippo has the hiccups: and other poems I totally made up (2009)
- The Biggest Burp Ever (2014)

Book List – Shadow Puppet Books

Shadow Night
Kay Chorao (2001)

After James thinks he sees the shadow of a monster, he calls Mama and Daddy, who calm his fears by showing him to use his hands to make other shadow shapes, including dogs, elephants, and alligators.

Making Shadow Puppets
Jill Bryant, Catherine Heard, and Laura Watson (2002)

In this Kids Can Do It title, kids discover the secret to creating traditional shadow puppets based on designs from around the world.

Shadow Puppets and Shadow Play
David Currell (2008)

Illustrating the work of some of the finest shadow players in the world, this book explains with clarity and precision the art of shadow puppetry, an art form increasingly used by professional companies and educational institutions.

The Art of Shadow Hands
Albert Almoznino (2002)

Over 70 illustrations of hand positions and actions to make lifelike animals and creatures.

Me and My Shadows - Shadow Puppet Fun for Kids of All Ages

Bud Banis PhD and Elizabeth Adams, 2013

Creative ways to do shadow puppetry using your hands and paper objects.

Book List – Native American Legends

The Story of Jumping Mouse

John Steptoe (1994)

A Native American legend retold and illustrated. The gifts of the Magic Frog and his own hopeful and unselfish spirit bring Jumping Mouse finally to the far-off land where no mouse goes hungry.

The First Strawberries - a Cherokee Story

Joseph Bruchac (1993)

A quarrel between the first man and the first woman is reconciled when the sun causes strawberries to grow out of the earth.

Iktomi and the Boulder

Paul Goble (1988)

A Plains Indian story, retold and illustrated. Iktomi, a Plains Indian trickster, attempts to defeat a boulder with the assistance of some bats in this story that explains why the Great Plains are covered with small stones (more titles in Iktomi series)

Between Earth and Sky:
Legends of Native American Sacred Places

Joseph Bruchac (author) and Thomas Locker (illustrator) (1996)

Retelling of various Native American legends that teaches a young boy that everything living and inanimate has its place, should be considered sacred, and given respect.

Miser on the Mountain:
A Nisqually Legend of Mount Rainier

Nancy Luenn (author) and Pier Morgan (illustrator) (1997)

Retelling of a traditional Pacific Northwest story of the man who climbs Mount Rainier to collect a valuable shell and discovers what is important in life.

Book List – Fables/Tall Tales/Multicultural

Ackamarackus:
Julius Lester's Sumptuously Silly Fantastically Funny Fables

Julius Lester (2001)

A collection of six original fables with morals both silly and serious.

Mice, Morals and Monkey Business:
Lively Lessons From Aesop's Fables

Christopher Wormell (2005)

Using colorful linoleum-block prints the author depicts the classic characters from Aesop's Fables.

Wisdom Tales From Around The World

Heather Forest (1996)

A collection of traditional stories from around the world, reflecting the cumulative wisdom of Sufi, Zen, Taoist, Buddhist, Jewish, Christian, African, and Native American cultures.

Book Of Virtues For Young People:
A Treasury Of Great Moral Stories
William J. Bennett (1997)

Well-known works including fables, folklore, fiction, drama, and more, by such authors as Aesop, Dickens, Tolstoy, Shakespeare, and Baldwin are presented to teach virtues, including compassion, courage, honesty, friendship, and faith.

Tall Tales of the Wild West:
A Humorous Collection of Cowboy Poems and Songs
Eric Ode (2007)

A collection of humorous poems about cowboys and the Old West, three of which are set to the tunes of popular songs.

Koi and the Kola Nuts
Verna Aardema (1999)

An African folktale in which the son of the chief must make his way in the world with only a sackful of kola nuts and the help of some creatures that he has treated with kindness.

Mufaro's Beautiful Daughters: an African Tale
John Steptoe (1987)

Murafo's two beautiful daughters, one bad tempered and one kind and sweet, go before the king, who is choosing a wife.

Backyard Theatre

by Olivia Sweeney

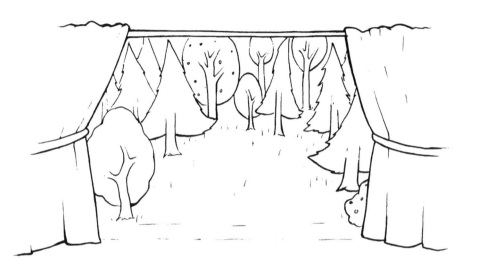

Backyard theater is a place to have fun, and be your own, zany self.

Imagination? Creativity? Improvisation? Bring it on! With backyard theatre, you can have loads of fun, without buying costumes, creating scripts, or stressing over performance day. I encourage you to make up your own story lines, use household materials for costumes, and stretch your minds to the fullest extent. There isn't a time limit - you could do this over a couple of days or just a few hours. It is all up to you!

Getting Started

You might want to do a couple games to get to know everyone and loosen up. One good game is called "All My Friends And

Neighbors". This game let's you tell things about yourself and learn things about others. Everyone, except one person takes off a shoe. All get into a circle, and put one shoe where you are standing. The person who did not take off a shoe goes into the middle of the circle. Let's pretend that person likes dogs. That person says, "I want to see all my friends and neighbors who like dogs. " Then everyone who likes dogs has to leave their shoe and go to a spot with another shoe. This gives the person in the middle a chance to go to a shoe too. One person will be left without a shoe spot and he or she goes into the middle and asks the next question. You can repeat this as many times as you want. To make it more fun, don't repeat questions.

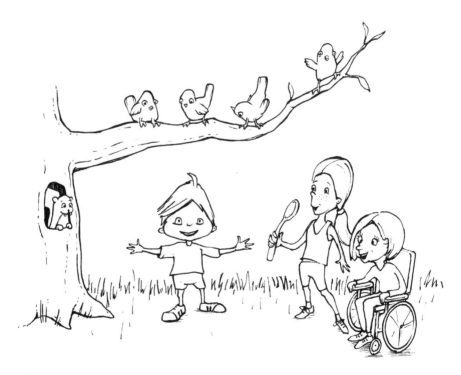

The Idea

Brainstorming

When you get your friends together you can think about what kind of performance you want to do. You may want to choose a topic and start a brainstorming session. Allow friends' ideas to expand the topic. Your ideas do not have to be totally developed. If you prefer, you may want to start an idea, and start to develop it on the spot, acting out what you think might happen.

Story Lining

Once you have a story idea, it is important to remember the structure of a good performance. You need a beginning, a middle, and an end, all clearly defined. In other words, a preface, a problem, a solution, and a conclusion.

So what is the problem? What can you do about the problem? What is the result? What is the big finish?

Using Your Space

Take advantage of your surroundings. That backyard play structure is not in your way. It is a castle defended by knights in shining armor. That tree is not blocking your path. It is a pillar that holds the keys of life at the top. A tree house could be a jungle city inhabited by elves. Whatever story line you choose to pursue, encourage everyone to use the entire area for the performance.

Creating costumes

If you wish to include costumes, think about what you need.

Keep it simple. Use what you already have. A tablecloth becomes a long skirt, a basket becomes a bonnet, and a scarf becomes an elaborate headdress. Ask everyone to use their imagination to create a costume for their character or work together. Imagination is important in creating costumes.

Audience

Who do you want your audience to be? Ask the kids to invite family members and neighbors so they will be surrounded by people who love them. And how will you let them know? Knock on doors or give out flyers. Just tell them when it is. Set up chairs and blankets for audience or ask them to bring their own.

Time for Performance

Finally, it's here! The day of the performance is an exciting day. Some people get nervous on performance day, and it is totally normal! Remember to stay in character! Take a deep breath, know the audience is rooting for you, and do your best. Remember, your performance is not supposed to be perfect or overly rehearsed. It is just about you having fun in a non-stressful environment. After the performance, have everyone take a bow while the audience claps. You deserve it!

Another Backyard Idea – Improvisation

Another fun thing to do with friends is improvisation or improv, for short. Improv means doing a scene without practicing it first. Instead of a script you just make things up as you go along. Since you do it with others you need to share the story and stage. One of the golden rules of improvisation is to always accept someone's suggestion. Improv is making up lines and actions on the spot, and that is difficult to do when someone is always saying "no". So if one person offers an idea, for example, "Let's go to the mall," if you say "yes", this scene can expand and grow. But if you say no, the scene can be cut off suddenly, with disappointing results. If your group decides on improvisation, remember to always be open to suggestions in the scene.

The Hitchhiker Game

This game can include four people, but it is different every time, and you can take turns. You nominate a driver, and that person pretends to be driving. The next person is the first hitchhiker. He or she asks to get into the car. This hitchhiker will pick a chosen characteristic, for example having the hiccups. Then the driver must pretend to have this characteristic too. The next hitchhiker gets into the car, and adds a new characteristic, maybe whistling. Both the driver and the first hitchhiker adopt the characteristic of the most recent person. Now they are hiccuping and whistling. Add the last hitchhiker and the final characteristic, perhaps, finger snapping. You have all four people in the car hiccuping, whistling and snapping their fingers. Finally, the hitchhikers leave the car in reverse order and the characteristic they brought to the car ends. Until only the driver is left.

In my life, theatre has had great importance to me. My mom always tells the story about how I came home from first grade one day and said, "Mom, I invited my friends over to have a performance!" That is how Olivia's Wish Theatre began. The stage is where I can find myself, and I love every minute of it. I hope you can find the same joy and freedom that I do.

Costumes and Props

by Marian Gerrits

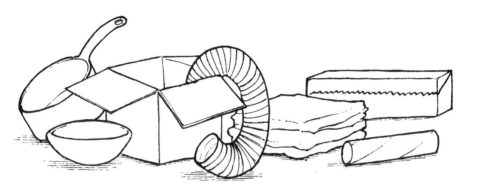

Costumes and props can be done by each participant or as a group. Imaginative use of items will add incredible dimension to any play. Below is a list of everyday items that can be used to make costumes. Remember to ask permission before you cut or mark anything permanently.

- Plastic bowls can be used for a hat, helmet, or shoulder pads.

- Pieces of cardboard can be used for many things like a curtain or backdrop.

- Table cloths can be used for bridal dresses, curtains, shawl, skirt, toga, sarong.

- Dryer vent flexible corrugated pipe (available at any hardware store) can be used for making robots, worms, or a tin man.

- Aluminum foil has many uses, some of which are bracelets, jewelry, shoes, robots, hats, antennae, and wands. It can also be used to cover cardboard to make robots.

- A towel can be a cape, rug, blanket, turban, or window curtain.

- Black plastic bags can be used to create witch costumes, vests, dresses, pants, skirts, capes, and window and theatre curtains.

- White plastic bags can be used to create angels and fairies, curtains, vests, dresses, hula skirts, fringe (like on a cowboy vest), ghosts, princesses, and head pieces by twisting them. You can use permanent markers, some paints, or cut, paste, or glue.

- Brown paper grocery sacks are good for shirts, vests, dresses (turn inside out if there is advertising on the bag). They can also be used for weaving or braiding strips, braided belts, and paper mache. Smaller bags can be used to make puppets.

- Newspaper can be used for braiding and paper mache, shaped hats, vests, or stuffing.

- Uses of an old white t-shirt are limited only to your imagination. Long-sleeved t-shirts can be head pieces, dresses or an apron. You can cut the sleeves off, cut fringe, and spray paint or dye them. Turn them inside out if there are words or logos on the shirts.

- Pillowcases can be used for dresses, vests, and other tops. See previous ideas for t-shirts above. Remember, don't cut things without permission!

- Props can include baskets, pots and pans, cardboard tubes from paper towels, toilet paper, or rug tubes, and boxes large and small. Check grocery stores, furniture stores, and stores that sell large appliances for big boxes, as well as cardboard that is usually sandwiched between layers of product when it is shipped. Think outside the box!

A Costume Exercise for Fun

Pebble Theatre is not only an opportunity for acting. Creative artists may wish to participate in costuming and design.

Invite a group of friends 9 years old (and older) to join you for a costume creation party. Ask each guest to bring a scissors to the party. Have a stack of newspapers (comic pages, advertising and news stories), a large stack of paper grocery bags, plastic bags of all shapes, colors and sizes, garbage bags, or the extra large leaf bags. Paper plates, rolls of toilet paper may be added to the mix. Provide tape of a variety of sizes and kinds. Ask for help if you need it!

Divide the guests into groups of two or three. Each group will be asked to choose from the stack of offerings to create a costume for one of their participants. The working group will also create a description of the costume -- what the costume is highlighting or used for or its unusual features. It can be funny, ridiculous, or serious. You may want to play music for the participants one by one to walk down the "runway", while the narrator speaks. You may wish to have adults be present for safety reasons or to become part of your audience.

Fun Icebreaker ideas

- Have each participant bring a hat to the first gathering. Each person must introduce him or herself by using voices and characteristics the hat might suggest.

- Have each participant bring an object from home that is easily recognizable for its purpose. Then ask each participant to use the object for a completely different imaginative purpose. For example, a toothbrush could be used to paint a house, or a large spoon can become a microphone.

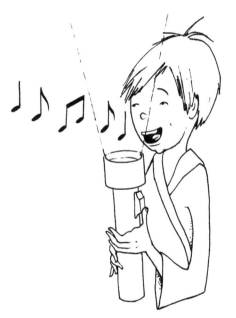

Stage Directions

Upstage Right	Upstage Center	Upstage Left
Stage Right	Stage Center	Stage Left
Downstage Right	Downstage Center	Downstage Left

Audience ~ Audience ~ Audience

When the actor stands on stage facing the audience, to his left is "**stage left**" and to his right is "**stage right**." Directly in the middle is "**center stage**." In front of the actor is "**down stage**." Behind the actor (at his back) is "**upstage**." It was named upstage in the early days of theatre because the back part of the stage was built up higher so the audience could see them better. Therefore it became known as "**upstage**." The area behind the back curtain is known as "**backstage**."

When the director gives you directions about movement regarding where to enter or exit, or when to sit or stand up it is called "**blocking**." If you are being given directions for moving with music, it is called "**choreography**." There is another use of the word "**blocking**." If an actor stands or moves in front of another actor, it is said that he was "**blocking**" that actor because no one can see the other actor. "**Blocking the audience**" refers to an actor who turns away from the audience blocking their view from the actors actions.

The word "**upstaging**" is also used if your character does something that distracts from another actor's significant moment. For instance, if an actor is giving a big speech (or a little statement) but you do something that draws attention away from that actor to yourself, such as fussing with your hair or moving around, that is called "**upstaging**."

A **prop** is something your character needs to add to the role. It may be a coat if it is cold, a book for a student, or a chair for an old man.

To **throw someone a line** means you prompt them with the line spoken before their line. To **run a scene** is to go through a scene from beginning to end. A **dress rehearsal** means to go through the entire play with costumes.

The audience is often referred to as the "**4th Wall**".

When the play is over and everything needs to be cleaned and put away, a term used is "**striking the stage**." Always ask everyone who has been a part of the production to help "**strike the stage**."

Moving Beyond the Basics

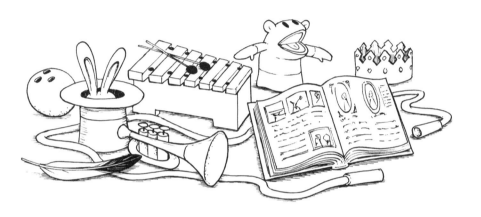

If you are a teenager or a seasoned actor try a few of the following activities! These are fun with friends, classmates, or an organization you enjoy.

Or are you a teacher who wants to include some imagination in your classroom? Give one or two of these ideas a try to bring fun into your classroom.

Notes:

Ice Breakers – Get Things Going

by Evan Powell

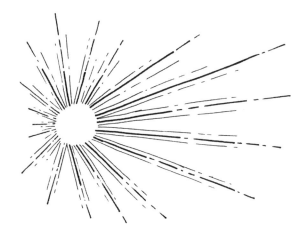

Ice breaker activities help people get to know each other better, have a little fun and often move the body around. In theater ice breakers take on new meaning when you need to plan for your role, pay attention to all that is happening around you, and be prepared in case someone forgets a line or enters without a prop. Quick thinking and focus are essential.

Alliteration Introduction

This is a nice game for everyone to get to know each other's names. Everyone gets into a circle and introduces themselves with a gesture and altering his name. An example would be, "I'm Cool Calvin" with a thumbs up sign or "I'm Loving Lacey" with a pat on the heart. The next player point to the first, repeats the previous player's name, attribute and gesture, and does something similar about himself and so on. The game ends when the gestures of the first player does all of the players' gestures, repeating their names and attributes.

Cartoony Cat & Mouse Chase

This is a very easy game to play. Two players chase each other around the room. The player being chased has to mime an obstacle for the other player to overcome. To keep the game fair and from going on, you can limit the amount of times the player can make obstacles before he is eventually caught.

Toboggan Buddies

This game needs lots of room and is easier to play on a smooth floor. For this physical team game, a group of 4 to 6 people sit in a line and wrap their legs around the person ahead of them. Place a line of masking tape at about 10 to 15 feet away. On Go, the team must race to the finish line but only using their hands and sliding. If the group breaks apart, they have to get back to together before crossing the finish line. If you want to add an element of excitement, have different teams timed to see who is the fastest.

Long Lost Friend

Pick one person to lead. To start out, everybody must walk around the room. On the leader's command, greet the closest person near you. Once you are done, walk around some more. From that point on, the leader will call how you will greet each other in a unique way. It could be as if they're greeting a long lost friend. It could be that they have to greet each other while laughing the entire time, or you could be acting like a head strong cowboy.

Mirror Mirror

For this game everyone needs to get in a circle. You and the person standing directly across from you has to start mirroring each other. Taking turns, the two mirroring each other must walk to the center of the circle and back to their place in the circle. After everyone has gone to the center and back, have the people in the circle start mirroring any person of their choosing. You can also have someone leave the room and have everyone in the circle choose one person to mimic. Be subtle about how you watch the leader so the guesser has to work at it. Once the person comes back in, he has to figure out who the group is mimicking.

Arrow, Baby, Angry Kitty

For this last game, have every one walk around the room. One person starts pantomiming that they are drawing and shooting an arrow at someone. Like a Kung Fu master, that player catches the arrow and shoots it at someone else. Once this has gone on for a while, have another person pantomime tossing a baby while creating the sound of a baby crying. Once the baby has been tossed around a bit, start tossing an angry cat to all the players. Make sure to add a distinct sound with everything you toss! As you get used to the game, you can toss whatever you want with it's own distinct sound to every player.

Notes:

Creating Improvisations

by Kendra Munroe

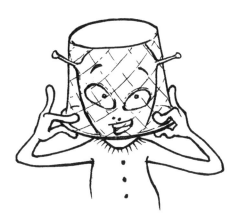

What is so special about improvisation theater? In fact, what is improvisation theater?

You've got your imagination, but you don't have a script? Perfect! Improvisation theater, more commonly known as improv, is a means of performing for others, or your own amusement, without having to worry about reading lines off of a pre-made script. No script is necessary because everything that is said or done is made up on the spot; it's pure impromptu imagination!

Basic improv rules:

An important rule of improv is never say 'no.' That may sound a bit harsh, but by saying 'no' during a scene it is similar to saying you do not like the other person's idea. Improv is about being able to express yourself in that moment without the worry of someone else saying 'no, I don't like your idea because I like mine better.' It is about working with a team and building trust among you and other improv players.

A second rule of improv is always help a team member when they are struggling during a scene. You must all work together as a cohesive entity for the scene to succeed. The best motto to have is 'All for one and one for all.' An example of a struggle would be if you sense the scene is falling apart. A possible solution would be to step in and add something interesting into the scene. You don't want to stop the scene completely because then your team member might feel bad. Work together; two heads are better than one and a full team of great ideas and willingness to help each other equals a successful scene.

A third rule of improv is 'do not be afraid to break down the 4th wall.' The 4th wall is that imaginary barrier actors have with the audience. When on stage we often are told to ignore the audience and pretend they are not there. Improv is the complete opposite. Audience participation can not only provide players with more material to work with during a scene, but it is also fun for the audience to feel like they are part of the team. Ask an audience member to participate in a sketch or scene. Ask the audience a question to assist in the setup of a scene. Improv is about breaking down any sort of barrier, including the 4th wall.

Obtaining ideas for the start of a scene:

What are prompts?

Prompts are something that help create a scene with the

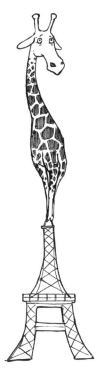

help of your other players or your audience. A prompt can provide the involved players ideas for characters, settings, and scene plots. The great thing about a prompt is it does not always have to make sense because it is up to the actors (players) to incorporate their interpretation of the audience answer into the scene.

Some examples of fun prompts would be...

- Where would you least likely find a giraffe?

- What would be a strange thing to wear on your head?

- What would be an unlikely name for a superhero?

The answers may vary every time you ask a difference person. Someone might say...

- The least likely place to find a giraffe would be on the top of the Eiffel Tower.

- A strange thing to wear on your head would be an octopus.

- An unlikely superhero name could be Captain Tuna Fish.

Question: Someone prompts you to do a scene from a well known book or movie. Take the Harry Potter series for instance. You

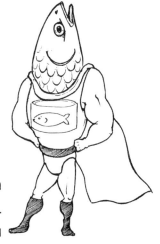

might ask, "would this be allowed during an improv scene even though it was not my original thought?"

Answer: You can include anything that is your interpretation if it helps to move the scene forward. You don't have to be the known Harry Potter characters or even have the well known locations in the books. You might just decide you are a wizard lost in Antarctica and you need to find a way home. Start with the basic idea and perform your own spin.

A few common improv games:

Freeze Tag -- Novice to Intermediate

You have a group of people together. Two or three of you go forward and start a scene (it can be anything!). At some point, usually after about 30 seconds, one of the people not involved in the scene yells, 'FREEZE!' The actors must immediately freeze in what every position they were in when they heard the freeze command. The person who yelled 'freeze' must then indicate to one of the actors currently 'frozen' to leave the scene and the person who called for the 'Freeze' must take exact position of the person who just left. Once the new player is in position he or she will create an entirely new scene until the next person yells 'Freeze. '

For example: Two people are doing a scene about finding an octopus in the ocean. Someone, not in the scene, yells 'FREEZE' and both actors freeze in their current position; one person with hands out like he or she is swimming while the other actor is in a crouched position trying hide from the octopus.

The person who yelled 'FREEZE' decides to take the place of the person who is pretending to swim. The person who just came into the scene decides the position of his or her arms is similar to that of a person who is brushing a very large horse, but they cannot reach the top of the horse's back. From this idea, the person starts this new scene involving a horse until someone again yells 'FREEZE.'

Half Life -- Intermediate to advanced

Half-Life is a game where one must race against the clock. First, designate one person to be the time keeper (preferably someone with a watch with a second hand, or a cell phone with a stopwatch). This person will keep track of the time and tell the players when to stop. You have six opportunities to run the same scene or as close as you can get the same scene. The first time you run the scene you have one minute to do so. The second time you run the same scene gets tricky because not only do you have to run the scene as close as to how it was during the first minute, this time you only have 30 seconds to complete the same scene. The third time you have 15 seconds, the forth 7 seconds, the fifth 3 seconds, and the sixth 1 second. You want to try your best to resolve the scene, but it's difficult because you don't know exactly how much time you may or may not have left during each time segment. Do not worry about fitting everything in each time. The scene will become shorter and shorter and you will find yourself forgetting pieces or talking faster.

For example: You and your fellow actors/teammates decide to do a scene about getting that giraffe out of the Eiffel Tower elevator and back to the zoo, but the giraffe keeps pressing the elevator buttons. (Remember: the scene is not decided before hand. You are given a prompt and an idea, but the creation of the scene is up to you as you go along). You will have one minute to play out this scene and return the giraffe to the zoo. The time keeper yells 'STOP' at the end of one minute. Now you have 30 seconds to recreate that exact scene (to the best of your abilities) and help get the giraffe out of the elevator. After the 30 seconds, your time is cut in half. Now do the scene in 15 seconds…7 seconds…3 seconds… 1 second. Once you get to the 1 second time, it is usually like a joke punch line. If you had been trying to get the giraffe out of the elevator the entire time, now say or do something opposite… "Wow! I love this new giraffe ride!"

Party Quirks -- Novice to Advanced

This is kind of like a guessing game for one of your team members. Decide who you want to be the 'party guests' (about 5 or 6 people) and who will be the 'party host.' 'Once you decide who will be the host, have them go somewhere so he or she will not be able to overhear what the rest of the team is saying. Next you want to decide a quirk for each party guest. The quirks are supposed to be an impression of a person, animal, or even an object. When all the 'party guests' have a quirk, the host is able to come back. Each 'guest' will arrive to the party one at a time (you can pretend you are ringing a doorbell or knocking so the 'host' has to answer the door). Be sure to give the 'host' at least a few seconds to talk with the newest 'guest' before the next 'guest' arrives to the party. This provides the host with some time to get to know each character. The 'host' will then try to guess who or what each person represents. As soon as the 'host' guesses the correct impression of a 'guest', the 'guest' will then bid farewell to the 'host' (remaining in character, of course) and leave the scene. Everyone applauds (other team members and audience) to show the 'host' guessed correctly.

For example: You have five people playing as guests and one person as the host. The person as the host goes somewhere so they cannot overhear each person's quirks. The five guests collectively decide on the quirks.

- 'Guest #1" is a flamingo.

- 'Guest #2' is a shark with a tooth ache.

- 'Guest #3' is the Easter Bunny.

- 'Guest #4' is a professional ice skater.

- 'Guest #5' is a lion tamer.

The host returns and 'Guest #1' enters the scene. This person is supposed to act like a flamingo; he or she might stand on one leg and flap his or her arms. Talk to the 'host' as if you were a flamingo… "Oh, your outfit is very dull. I prefer brighter colors myself…Oh, I see you like standing on two legs; I find standing just one more comfortable." (You do not want to make it too easy for the 'host' to guess.)

'Guest #2' enters with his/her hands together on top of their head like a fin, "I was just eating some fish and it must have been really really stale because when I bit into it…ow."

'**Guest #3**' hops into the scene. "Hello, I'm so hoppy to see you…oh, is that chocolate and deviled eggs?"

'**Guest #4**' glides into the scene, greets host, and does a spin then glides away to other 'guests. '

'**Guest #5**' charges into the scene. "It's great to see you again. Down kitty!" Guest yells while pretending to keep host at a distance while using an imaginary chair and whip.

The host can guess a character right away or they can observe a couple more minutes. If the 'host' wants to talk to a guest again before deciding what he or she might be, that is encouraged. When all of the characters have been guessed the game is over.

"Do-Run-Run" -- Novice-Intermediate

This is a good acting warm-up or cool down for two or more people. It is a musical improv game that combines chanting with rhyming. The rhyming pattern is A-A-B-B-B. Usually the first and second parts of the chant (the two A parts) are eight or nine syllables. The third, fourth, and fifth parts (the three B parts) are usually four to five syllables. Each part is chanted by a different person. It is often easiest if all of the players are in a circle so the chant continues without a pause. Try to go for as long as you can without someone messing up the pattern or not being able to continue on with the rhyming.

This example is for six people (note the words in italics are the parts of the chant, the actors change each time) - you may want to change the rhythm or chant for your particular group:

- **Actor #1** (pattern A): *"I went to the park the other day…"*

- **Everyone**: "A-do-run-run-run-ah-do-run-run"

- **Actor #2** (pattern A): *"And my mom said that was okay…"*

- **Everyone**: "Ah-do-bah-do-yeah!"

- **Actor #3** (pattern B): *"I saw a mouse!"*

- **Everyone**: "Ah-do-bah-do-yeah!"

- **Actor #4** (pattern B): *"It was wearing a blouse!"*

- **Everyone**: "Ah-do-bah-do-yeah!"

- **Actor #5** (pattern B): *"It's as big as my house!"*

- **Everyone**: "Ah-do-run-run-run-ah-do-run-run"

- **Actor #6** (pattern A): *"I was scared so I climbed a tree."*

- **Everyone**: "Ah-do-run-run-run-ah-do-run-run"

- **Actor #1** (pattern A): *"I really hoped that mouse didn't see."*

- **Everyone**: "Ah-do-bah-do-yeah!"

- **Actor #2** (pattern B): *"I see a lake!"*

- **Everyone**: "Ah-do-bah-do-yeah!"

- **Actor #3** (pattern B): *"I could eat some cake!"*

- **Everyone**: "Ah-do-bah-do-yeah!"

- **Actor #4** (pattern B): *"Is that a snake?!?"*

- **Everyone**: "Ah-do-run-run-run-ah-do-run-run"

- The song continues following the same A-A-B-B-B pattern.

Pillars -- Intermediate

This is a game usually played by four people. Two players are each a "pillar" and the remaining two players are the actors. Each actor has a designated "pillar" to provide words, sound effects, or ideas for the scene. The actors are able to move around during the scene, however the pillars are to be stationary like a stone pillar.

The two actors begin a scene. Every once in a while they utilize their "pillar" to fill-in an idea.

For Example: One of the actors begins a scene about two friends on a sail boat in the middle of Pacific Ocean. The two friends are on a trip to find the world's largest Tuna Fish.

During the scene one of the actors might say something like, "we need to have strong equipment to hold such a large fish. Perhaps if we get lots of…" Instead of finishing the sentence yourself, you tap your "pillar's" shoulder to provide them a cue to fill in the rest of your sentence. So the "pillar" might say, "purple worms covered in green sparkles. "The actor will then repeat the sentence he or she just said, this time inserting what the "pillar" has said into the original sentence. The rest of the scene continues with each actor using his or her "pillar" to fill pieces of sentences now and then.

Caution: As part of the game, the actor must try to use whatever comes out of the "pillar's" mouth. So if the "pillar" cannot think of anything to say then he or she merely laughs. The actor must incorporate the laughter into the part of the previous sentence. It's improv, so be prepared for the unpredictability of your "pillars."

Props -- Intermediate-Advanced

Have everyone in your group find one strange item at home that can be used as a prop (a few examples could be: a swimming noodle, a blanket, an empty basket, an egg beater, etc.). You can either use the props to create an entire scene or you can have each person take turns creating advertisements for a new invention, creation, or discovery. Remember to use your imagination, the prop you choose is no longer the common household item…make it represent something completely different. Take the basket for example: it could be an alien head-dress, it could be the world's worse umbrella, it could be a bonnet from the pioneer days, it could be the collar a dog uses when delivering newspapers…there is no limit to your imagination!

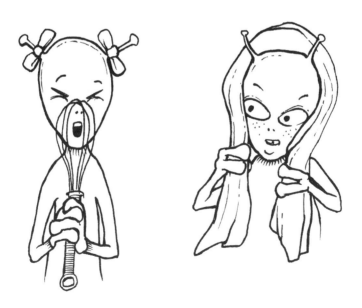

Other forms of improv:

Long-form -- Also known as The Harold

Long-form improv is considered to be a more advanced practice of improv. It is not made up of separate games. It is set up closer to that of an actual stage play. There is a beginning, a middle, and an end. You have various scenes that you progress though in order to complete the act; the entire thing can last 15 to 30 minutes. Long-form works best with a strong sense of teamwork.

The biggest difference between long-form and an actual stage play is the fact that you have various scenes (each one possibly involving different people or settings) to work from. You may start out with one scene, but once the scene starts to flounder than another player will 'wipe' the scene by running in front of the players. When the scene is 'wiped' then a new scene begins using different actors. The process continues for three to four different scenes. After a 'wipe' you do not need to start a brand new scene; return to one of the already established scenes to pick up where you left off or act as though a time progression has happened (thus continuing the scene as if it were five hours later). By the end of the Long-form all of your established scenes should be able to end appropriately.

Commedia dell'Arte:

This is a type of Italian improv which originated around the 16th century. Commedia dell'Arte uses specific characters (stock characters) throughout each performance. Even though the scenes are different each time they are performed, the stock characters used always had the same personality. The audience would always be able to tell which character was which by the masks worn by the actors.

Examples of some stock characters and their masks:

- **Arlecchino**: The harlequin. A zany (fool) who is known for being a servant and a trickster. His mask usually has a giant wart/zit on the forehead and a large nose.

- **Il Capitano**: This character often brags of his adventures and soldier like qualities. However when true danger arises, Il Capitano is the first one to flee from the danger. Many times this mask will have a large mustache and a large nose.

- **Leandro**: The lover. He jumps into love too easily and will do anything for that love even if it means putting himself in some pretty silly situations. The mask is usually that of a young man. It does not have as many wrinkles as many of the other male character masks.

- **Pantelone**: The miser. He is an old, cranky character who only really cares about money. His mask usually has a longer pointed noise and lots of wrinkles.

- **Truffeldino**: He is a glutton and loves to play tricks on others. His one true love is Smeraldina whom Truffeldino loves to spoil. This mask often has large apple like cheeks to portray Truffeldino's gluttonous mannerisms.

There are many more Commedia dell'Arte characters. If you are interested in learning more about Commedia dell'Arte or more about other forms of improv theatre… check out your local library for books on improv history and more improv game ideas.

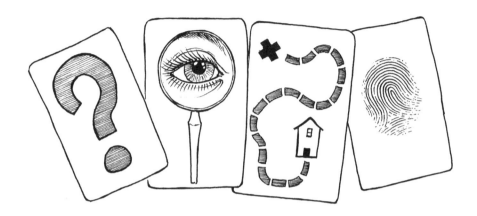

Creating Mystery Theatre

What is Mystery Theatre?

Mystery Theatre can be considered a party game. You can perform this type of theatre during your birthday party or just a fun gathering of friends on a rainy day. It is a type of theatre that combines the use of a script and style of long-form improv. Each person involved is a different character and you work through the script, broken down into specific sections, in order to figure out a whodunit type mystery.

Mystery Theatre is typically performed by young people and adults due to the themes and structure. Many times, the rules, guidelines, and structure of this type of theatre or game are too difficult for younger children to understand. It is heavily based on reading the script as the story line progresses and knowing what type of information to disclose at which times. In Mystery Theatre, the people participating are not given the script until the very last minute; there is no time to rehearse your lines.

Similar to improv theatre, you will have to think on your feet when another player talks to you or accuses you of something. You may need to use those quick thinking skills to provide an explanation or answer. However, unlike improv you will have a script in front of you at all times and you are able to reference back to the approved sections as needed throughout the mystery in order to refute the accusation.

How to create your own mystery:
Many times you can find a box mystery in a store, but why spend money when you can create your own personal mystery? Base the mystery on something you know. A lot of inspiration comes from books, movies, other plays, personal experiences, etc.

If you create your own mystery, then you are able to add a personal spin to the game; which in turn can make it more meaningful for you and your friends.

One thing is for sure when creating your own mystery theatre game; you must be very organized during the creation process. Without good organization, it is easy to get lost and lose bits of needed information. A few tips for staying organized might include keeping all information in a binder with separate sections for characters, settings, plots, clues, etc; creating separate documents on the computer for characters, clues, etc; keeping all information in one note book, but color coding each category/section using different colored pens so you don't confuse your character information with your clue information.

When creating a mystery there are some questions you need to answer:

- How many characters?
- What personalities do the characters have?
- Do the characters have any secrets? And what are the secrets?
- What kind of mystery do the characters need to solve or for what purpose did all of these characters need to be gathered in one place?
- What bits of information should each character have about other characters?
- What is the idea or plot?
- Was something stolen? Something lost? Did something strange happen?
- What might the clues be? (treasure maps, foot/fingerprints, etc)

A sample mystery: "The Case of the Missing School Mascot"

- What kinds of questions go through your mind when you read that title?
- Who stole the mascot?
- What does the mascot look like? Was the mascot an animal or a costume?
- Where was the mascot last seen?

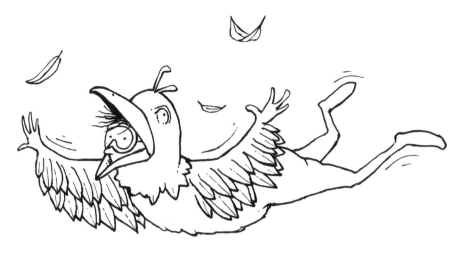

- Who were the last person/people to see the mascot?

- Who knew where the mascot was located?

- Who had the motive to steal the mascot? And what could be a possible motive?

- To answer our questions let's say…

- Jim Nasium stole the mascot.

- The mascot was a giant bird costume with feathers hanging down the arms to look like wings.

- The mascot bird costume was last seen in the storage closet under the bleachers.

- The last people to see the mascot costume were Jim Nasium, Cam Estry, Inga Lishe, Al Jabrah, Ima Bookworm, and Historia Past.

- Jim Nasium, Inga Lishe, Al Jabrah, and Historia Past knew the location of the mascot costume.

- Jim Nasium was hoping the school would purchase

a new costume if the old one was stolen. Cam Estry wanted to use the feathers on the costume for science experiments. Inga Lishe was terrified of birds and did not want to see the costume during games. Al Jabrah wanted to play a prank on his students and thought stealing the mascot costume would be funny. Ima Bookworm did not think it was an accurate representation of the glorious Thunderbird and often vocalized how she wished the costume would disappear. Historia Past was bitter she was not the mascot when she was in school.

With those few questions you were able to answer who the involved characters were, what the mystery was, the motives of each character, the location of the mystery, and whodunit!

Build from each set of answers. Keep asking yourself questions. After a few rounds of asking yourself questions and then answering those questions putting together the last details of the mystery should be simple.

Then break down your information into 3 to 4 sections. Divide bits of character insight and clues into each of the sections for each character.

The best way to figure out if your mystery has any kinks to work out is to gather your friends together to play out the mystery. Once you figure out where the weaknesses are, make note and fix it so the next time you do the mystery with a different group of friends then it will run more smoothly.

One problem with mystery theatre is the mystery can only be played one time per group of friends. This is because people who participate in the same mystery would already know the outcome of the mystery. On the other hand, you can adapt your game to become a full length play. All you would have to do is practice the mystery a few times with your friends, find an audience to watch, and then have the audience guess whodunit at the end of the play.

Thank you!

If you have read all or any part of this little book, *we thank you!*
Now comes the exciting part.

When you put your voice,
your imagination,
your acting,
your costumes, and

Your Spin

on any of these ideas,
you will be creating that magic,
that magic that is known as

Theatre!

So, now - Go!
Create your very own Pebble Theatre!
Good Luck or as we say in the theatre ...

Break a Leg

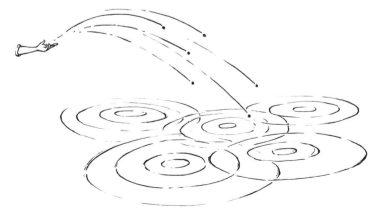

Biographies

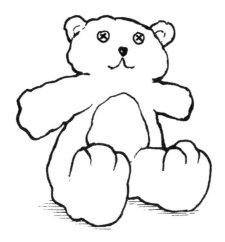

Donna E. Nylander

Donna, a teacher, a founder and director of the Ellensburg Children's Musical Theatre, began telling and writing stories for children many years ago. She prefers to write stories and plays that have educational and meaningful topics while using magic and music to enhance the experiences of the participant. She created Pebble Theatre as a special summer program to encourage young people to create their own stories, plays, costumes and props from their surroundings. In today's world filled with technology and instant awe, she enjoys the young person who ponders, imagines, creates, interacts, and is willing to share an artistic endeavor with others. Plays she created include subjects as varied as bullying, The Berlin Wall, Lewis and Clark, honoring the environment, Leonardo De Vince, Neil Armstrong, Helen Keller, Malala, friendships, and the value of music, color and laughter in our lives.

Marian Gerrits

Marian says that three women took her under their wing: Marge Corman, Val Lister, and Donna Nylander. These ladies gave her permission to do whatever she could dream. Her love of old things and new opportunities came at the right time for her to feel part of a community. Together with Ellensburg Children's Musical Theatre (EMCT), Frontier Village, and Moments to Remember a forty-year friendship was formed. Marian will never forget the faces of kids who would become street vendors, angels, shepherds. She said, "These events are what makes Ellensburg my home town." Marian is a founder of EMCT, and the creator of the Streets of Bethlehem for Moments to Remember.

Debbie Vosburgh

From the age of eight Debbie had her fingers on a typewriter keyboard, and later computers. Her skill and speed were a part of almost every job she has held, from office manager to executive assistant, and most recently, medical transcription. In 2001 she was gifted with meeting Donna Nylander, who was looking for a typist/editor for her Ellensburg Children's Musical Theatre scripts. Seven scripts and fourteen years later the two have become the dearest of friends. Debbie was honored to be asked to help with the transcription, formatting, and editing of the early drafts of this book.

Nomi Pearce

Nomi's earliest memories of theatre are in the backyard with friends and cousins. After a quick story development her mom would be finding costumes and baking brownies. Generous neighbors would come to the shows. Nomi danced and choreographed in college. She was invited to choreograph and dance in one of her Mom's Ellensburg Children's Musical Theatre productions. When she became a mom, she led a backyard theatre camp for her seven year old daughter and her friends "Olivia's Wish Theatre." After some games and improvisation activities six kids were given a few props and they developed their own story. At the end of the camp parents gathered for a potluck and a show. Today Nomi coordinates a culture and language outreach program at Willamette University. She is grateful to her husband who knows the importance of tea.

Olivia Sweeney

Olivia lives in rainy Salem, Oregon. She has always been involved in performing arts, whether it is singing at home, backyard theatre, choir, or camps. She participates in Children's Educational Theatre, an annual five-week intensive program in the summer, where she enjoys classes such as monologues, dance, musical theatre, flash mob, and Commedia dell'Arte. She performed in school plays since first grade, and she studies several styles of dance. Olivia is grateful that Heritage School emphasized both visual and performing arts, and that she was born into a family that lives artfully. Olivia loves to sing, dance, and spend time with her friends.

Kendra Munroe

Kendra lives in western Massachusetts, where she works as an occupational therapist (which she loves!) at a local hospital. She has been involved in the theatre arts from a young age both on stage and behind the scenes. Her involvement in theatre started with performing small roles for her church Christmas pageants and from there she began participating in various high school and community shows. Once in college, she became involved in two different college improv troupes. Theatre has helped Kendra become more confident and has helped her think on her feet during tough situations; after all, "…all the world's a stage!"

Evan Powell

Evan started out in the theatre at a very young age. His first performance was in a children's play at the age of 11. Upon graduation he was honored with an Excellence in Drama award by Ellensburg High School. He went on to pursue a degree at Central Washington University, graduating with a BA in Theatre. Evan is a licensed massage practitioner and is currently studying holistic healing.

Justin Gibbens

Thirty-some odd years ago when he first began moving graphite on paper, Justin was rendering the childhood standards: dinosaurs, creepy crawlers, and other freakish fauna. Not much has changed in three decades. Trained in both scientific illustration and traditional Chinese painting, Gibbens uses this skill set in his subversive zoological drawings. He is a founding member of PUNCH Gallery, an artist-run gallery located in Seattle, Washington. Gibbens was the recipient of a 2006 Pollock-Krasner Foundation Award and a 2008 Artist Trust Fellowship Award. He has shown his artwork nationally and internationally. He lives in rural Thorp, Washington.

Josephine Yaba Camarillo

Josephine is the Children's and Young Adult Librarian at the Ellensburg Public Library. She has been in her position since

Fall 2000. She enjoys working with children and families at the library and the community, performing story time and hosting fun library events. She is a dedicated member of the Ellensburg Children's Musical Theatre with Spring productions, holiday performances, and special engagements. She is an advocate for reading, early literacy, and performing arts for kids. She is also an avid runner, and is assistant cross country coach for Ellensburg High School. She enjoys eating pizza tossed by her wonderful husband Chef KC. But foremost, she is grateful for the love, encouragement, and support from Donna Nylander, introducing Josephine to this beautiful place called Ellensburg and helping her call it home.

Bill Sweeney
After graduating from Central Washington University with a graphic design degree, Bill started his own business called Doggone Design. His favorite client eventually became his wife, though the print job never panned out. An opportunity to move to Oregon was too good to pass up and now he combines design and data for the Oregon State Legislature. He has contributed his talents to ECMT productions through extraordinary props and publicity materials. He illustrated, designed and published The Teddy Bear's First Christmas by Donna Nylander. Occasionally he designs and builds custom screen doors. Everyday he makes his wife a cup of tea before waking her. He dreams of sailing the big water.

The End - It's a wrap

Pebble Theatre Certificate

_____

(name)

is an important member of Pebble Theatre

for the contribution of

_____

_____

Date